EAT FAT COOKBOOK
50 GET THIN MEALS

Break the Cycle of Cravings, Intense Hunger and Overeating with Eat Fat Get Thin Diet

Brian Perry

Table of Contents

Introduction

This book contains proven steps and strategies on how to eat fat and still get thin, and eliminate cravings and extreme hunger through the Eat Fat, Get Thin Diet. This breakthrough will change everything you have ever thought were true when it comes to eating fat. If you haven't heard of yet, eating fat will not make you gain weight or is not the root cause of different heart ailments. It is actually the exact opposite. If you want to eliminate overeating, break the cycles of intense cravings, and ultimately get thin then eat fat. Science has this to back up.

What you are about to read is an overview of the said diet and 50 get thin recipes you will surely be amazed to know and practice preparing. In the duration of following this diet, make sure to regularly track your body measurements, your blood pressure and cholesterol levels, and how much hours of sleep and physical activity you have done. This way, you will immediately know that the diet is really working for you and suits your body and lifestyle best.

The single best thing that you can do for your health is to know what you are putting in your body. In order to achieve a healthy body and longer life is to eat more fat. Yes, you heard it right. Eat more fat in order to lose weight, feel good about yourself, and prevent diseases.

You sure are aware of the dangers of having too much sugar in your diet, and you may be asking yourself what to eat now. The answer is fat. This 3 letter word no longer spells danger in one's health. Science has revealed that dietary fat will not cause weight gain if that is what you are worrying about. The advice you get about fat contributing to wider waistlines is scientifically incorrect. If you are thrilled to know more about this, read on and get to know different recipes you can make.

Thanks for purchasing this book. I hope you enjoy it.

Chapter 1: The Eat Fat Get Thin Diet – An Overview

Hard science has already threw light on the idea that high fat diet is the root cause of having heart diseases. Did you know that even saturated fats are no longer on the list of "this is bad for you" category? Eggs are also back! The reality is that the more fat you eat, the more you will lose weight and experiences better body functions. Now is the perfect time to rethink of your fear of fat. Instead, stop eating sugar and refined carbohydrates. And eat, yes, that yummy, filling, creamy, but not fattening kind of fat.

Many people are misled of the dietary guidelines stating that one should eat less fat and more carbohydrates that in the end, only leads to higher rates of diabetes and obesity. This said, it only means that the old way is not working. So what is so special about this diet program? Why does it work powerfully in helping you shed pounds, eliminate cravings, and reverse diseases? Take note of the following:

It takes advantage of the power of real, whole food –food are not only calories but given the right information, it is easy to program your body for optimal health. Food does not only fill the body, but it is also considered to be a potent medicine provided that you fuel the body with the right kinds of food and get rid of the bad foodstuff. When you say real food, it should comprise of whole, fresh produce. Everything else outside that scope is not considered food. Take note, the leading cause of obesity and diabetes in the world is because of high calorie and processed food. They are not only sugar laden but are also deficient in vital nutrients.

It cools down body inflammation – inflammation is the body's reaction to fight off bacteria and heal wounds. And by wounds we mean not just the cuts and sprained ankles, but those that are hidden and does not hurt. This is the immune system's way of fighting off stress, toxins, bad food, and even those low grade infections. Keep in mind, what causes insulin resistance comes from anything that causes inflammation. Insulin resistance generates the fat in your midsection and sabotages your weight loss efforts. The primary food triggering inflammation are gluten and dairy food. That is why they need to be eliminated when you are into this diet program.

It shuts your fat storage hormone also known as insulin – it is the insulin that instructs the body to pack on fat. It is discharged from the pancreas the moment you eat sugary food or carbohydrates containing sugar. Remember, food containing fructose, once absorbed by the stomach, goes straight to the liver triggering the production of fat, setting up a cascade of biochemical changes and significantly increasing diabetes and insulin resistance. What makes you fat is definitely too much insulin in the body all because of excessive consumption of sugar, carbohydrates, and animal protein. On the other hand, when you eat fat, the body does not produce insulin.

It switches off food cravings – dietary fat turns off food cravings making it way easier to regulate your appetite. When you eat fat, a chain reaction triggers both in the brain and body stopping the vicious cycle of cravings and overeating.

It makes you happy – did you know that fat is the key ingredient for proper nerve and brain functioning? Therefore, this kind of diet plan will make you happy as the good fats such as eggs and butter are now back in the menu. All you have to do is to steer clear of the bad stuff (everything that has sugar or turned into sugar once consumed by the body), and put in the good and healthy fats.

What You Will Eat

The following is a list of approved food:

- Consume only healthy fats such as olive oil, avocado, nuts, and seeds.
- A small amount of starchy vegetables such as sweet potatoes, parsnips, and squash are fine, but do not eat grains.
- Some of the low starch vegetables that you may consume at any amount include arugula, artichokes, asparagus, bell peppers, broccoli, Brussels sprouts, cabbage, cauliflower, celery, chives, collard greens, dandelion, eggplant, garlic, ginger, green beans, jalapenos, kale, lettuce, mushrooms, onions, radish, shallots, spinach, tomatoes, watercress and zucchini.
- When it comes to fruits, you should limit intake from 1 to 1 /2 cup per day of watermelon, lemons, berries, kiwi, and pomegranate.
- Some of the approved condiments include, apple cider vinegar, balsamic vinegar, sea salt, almond

flour, coconut flour, gluten free tamari, Dijon mustard, chicken and vegetable stocks, black peppercorns, and different herbs and spices such as onion, basil, parsley, cumin, oregano, cayenne pepper, chili powder, thyme, cinnamon, turmeric, sage, coriander, cardamom, ginger, paprika, and rosemary.

Food to Avoid

- All processed meats such as hotdog, bacon, salami, and canned meats among others.
- Grains, bread, and pasta.
- Gluten food.
- Soy sauce and soup mixes.
- Dairy except clarified butter.
- Artificial sweeteners.
- Alcohol.
- Refined vegetable oils such as canola oil, corn, safflower, sunflower, and soy.
- Fruits except for the ones listed above.

Chapter 2 – Healthy Breakfast Options

Recipe #1 - Strawberry, Berries and Mint Salad + Lemon Bars with Almonds Smoothie

Ingredients:

- 2 pieces, large mint leaves, julienned
- ¼ pound fresh strawberries, halved
- 1 teaspoon fresh blueberries
- 1 teaspoon fresh cranberries
- 1 teaspoon fresh raspberries
- 1 teaspoon lime juice, freshly squeezed
- ½ teaspoon date sugar, divided

Directions:

1. Place fruits into salad bowl. Toss to combine.
2. Place equal portions into bowls.
3. Just before eating, drizzle lime juice and date sugar on top. Serve immediately.

Lemon Bars with Almonds Smoothie

Ingredients:

- 1 large lemon, freshly juiced
- 1 cup almond slivers, freshly toasted

- 1 cup icy water

Directions:

1. Process all ingredients in blender until smooth. Pour equal portions into glasses. Serve.

Recipe #2 - Fresh Tomato Salad + Strawberry Smoothie Laced with Chia Seeds

Ingredients:

- 1 teaspoon capers in brine
- ½ pound tomatoes, chopped
- ¼ cup fresh basil leaves, minced

For the Dressing

- 3 teaspoons balsamic vinegar
- 3 teaspoons extra virgin olive oil
- 1 teaspoon maple syrup
- pinch of sea salt
- pinch of white pepper

Directions:

1. Pour dressing ingredients into small bottle with tight fitting lid. Seal and shake bottle until salt and sugar dissolves.
2. Place remaining ingredients into salad bowl; drizzle in dressing. Toss to combine.
3. Place equal portions into bowls. Serve immediately.

Strawberry Smoothie Laced with Chia Seeds

Ingredients:

- 1 cup frozen strawberries, quartered

- 1 cup icy water
- ½ cup watermelon, quartered
- 1 vanilla pod, discard pod
- 1 tablespoon chia seeds

Directions:

1. Process all ingredients in blender until smooth.
2. Pour equal portions into glasses. Serve.

Recipe #3 - Tofu Spinach Quiche + Berry Flavored Coconut Water

Ingredients:

- 8 oz extra firm tofu, drained and rinsed
- 2 ½ tablespoons non-dairy milk
- 1 onion, diced
- 1 garlic clove, minced
- 2 cups spinach, rinsed
- ½ cup Cheddar cheese
- ¼ cup Swiss cheese
- 1 vegetarian mini pie crust
- ¼ teaspoon sea salt

Directions:

1. Set the oven to 350 degrees F.
2. Blend the tofu and milk in a food processor. Season with salt and pepper.
3. Combine the cheeses, onion, spinach, garlic, and milk-tofu mixture in a bowl. Pour into the pie crust.
4. Bake for 15 minutes, or until heated through.
5. Set on a cooling rack for 5 minutes. Slice and serve.

Berry Flavored Coconut Water

Ingredients:

- 4 cups filtered water
- 2 cup fresh coconut water, unsweetened

- 1 cup frozen blueberries, unthawed
- 1 cup frozen blackberries and cranberries, unthawed

Directions:

1. Place ingredients into large pitcher. Secure lid. Chill in fridge for at least 5 hours prior to serving.
2. Using a muddler, stir drink, bruising some of the fruits to release more flavor. Strain infusions directly into tall glasses. Serve.

Recipe #4 - Berry Pancakes

Ingredients:

- ½ cup whole wheat flour
- ½ cup non-dairy milk
- 1 tablespoon olive oil
- 1 ½ tablespoons maple syrup
- ¼ cup berries
- ½ tablespoon baking powder
- 1/8 teaspoon sea salt

Directions:

1. Combine the flour, baking powder, and salt in a bowl.
2. Combine the milk, maple syrup, and canola oil in another bowl.
3. Mix the milk mixture into the flour mixture until just combined. Fold in the berries.
4. Heat a non-stick skillet over medium high flame. Ladle the batter into the skillet and cook for 2 minutes per side, or until golden. Repeat with the remaining batter.
5. Stack on a plate and serve.

Recipe #5 - Red Salad + Cilantro, Cucumber and Lime Flavored Water

Ingredients:

- 1 cup red leaf lettuce, torn
- 1 cup red oak lettuce, torn
- ½ cup red cherry tomatoes, quartered
- ¼ cup fresh raspberries

For the Dressing

- 3 teaspoons lemon juice, freshly squeezed
- 1 teaspoon extra virgin olive oil
- 1 teaspoon English or Russian (hot) mustard
- pinch of sea salt
- pinch of white pepper

Directions:

1. Pour dressing ingredients into small bottle with tight fitting lid. Seal and shake bottle until dressing emulsifies.
2. Place remaining ingredients into salad bowl; drizzle in dressing. Toss to combine. Place equal portions into bowls. Serve immediately.

Cilantro, Cucumber and Lime Flavored Water

Ingredients:

- 6 cups filtered water
- 2 cucumber, cubed
- 2 lime, sliced into wedges
- 1 fresh cilantro

Directions:

1. Place ingredients into large pitcher. Secure lid. Chill in fridge for at least 5 hours prior to serving.
2. Using a muddler, stir drink, bruising some of the fruits to release more flavor. Strain infusions directly into tall glasses. Serve.

Recipe #6 - Avocado and Tomato Salad on Tangy Vinaigrette

Ingredients:

- 3 ripe tomatoes, diced
- ½ ripe avocado, diced
- ½ iceberg lettuce, torn

For the Dressing

- 3 teaspoons extra virgin olive oil
- 3 teaspoons apple cider vinegar
- 1 Dijon mustard
- ½ teaspoons garlic powder
- ⅛ teaspoons white pepper
- ⅛ cup fresh chives, minced
- pinch of sea salt

Directions:

1. Pour dressing ingredients into small bottle with tight fitting lid. Seal and shake bottle until salt and sugar dissolves.
2. Place remaining ingredients into salad bowl; drizzle in dressing. Toss to combine. Place equal portions into bowls. Serve immediately

Recipe #7 - Veggie Hash Browns

Ingredients:

- ½ tablespoon olive oil
- 1 small red-skinned potato, grated
- 1 small sweet potato, grated
- 1 small carrot, grated
- 1 small zucchini, grated
- 1 small yellow summer squash, , grated
- ¼ cup minced red onion
- ¼ cup minced red bell pepper
- ¼ tsp paprika
- ¼ tsp garlic powder
- ¼ tsp sea salt
- 1/8 tsp freshly ground black pepper

Directions:

1. Combine the grated vegetables in a colander. Squeeze excess moisture. Transfer to a bowl.
2. Add the remaining ingredients, except olive oil, to the grated veggie mixture. Mix well.
3. Place a non-stick skillet over medium high flame and heat the olive oil.
4. Add the veggie mixture and flatten out. Pack firmly with a spatula and cook for 5 minutes, undisturbed, over medium flame.
5. Flip over and cook for an additional five to eight minutes, undisturbed, until crisp and golden brown. Serve hot.

Recipe #8 - Cashew Nut Jelly with Citrus Salad, Vegan

Ingredients:

- cashew nut jelly
- 2 cups cashew milk, unsweetened
- 2 cups water
- 2 pouches unflavored gelatin
- 2 teaspoons palm sugar, crumbled
- ½ teaspoons vanilla extract
- coconut oil for greasing

Fruit salad

- 2 mandarin oranges, pulp only
- 1 grapefruit, pulp only, torn into bite-sized pieces
- 1 pomelo, pulp only, torn into bite-sized pieces
- ½ cup roasted cashew nuts, chopped

Directions:

1. Lightly grease an 8" x 8" glass baking dish with coconut oil. Except for vanilla extract, combine remaining almond jelly ingredients in saucepan set over medium heat; stir until gelatin dissolves. Simmer while stirring continuously.
2. Gelatin is done when it sticks to the back of the spoon. Turn off heat immediately. Stir in vanilla extract.

3. Carefully pour gelatin into prepared baking dish. Cool completely to room temperature before sealing dish with saran wrap. Chill well before slicing into bite-sized cubes.
4. To make fruit salad: except for cashew nuts, place remaining ingredients into bowl; add in sliced gelatin. Toss gently to combine.
5. Ladle equal portions into bowls; garnish with cashew nuts. Serve.

Recipe #9 - Flax Milk Jelly with Berries, Vegan

Ingredients:

- flax milk jelly
- 2 cups flax milk, unsweetened
- 2 cups water
- 2 pouches unflavored gelatin
- 2 teaspoons palm sugar, crumbled
- ½ teaspoon vanilla extract
- coconut oil for greasing

Berry salad

- 1 tablespoon flax seeds, toasted
- 1 cup frozen strawberries, thawed
- 1 cup frozen blackberries, thawed
- ½ cup frozen blueberries, thawed
- ½ cup frozen raspberries, thawed

Directions:

1. To make flax milk jelly: very lightly grease an 8" x 8" glass baking dish with coconut oil. Except for vanilla essence, combine remaining ingredients in saucepan set over medium heat; stir until gelatin dissolves. Simmer while stirring continuously.
2. Gelatin is done when it sticks to the back of the spoon. Turn off heat immediately. Stir in vanilla essence.

3. Carefully pour gelatin into prepared baking dish. Cool completely to room temperature before sealing dish with saran wrap. Chill well before slicing into bite-sized cubes.
4. To make berry salad: except for flax seeds, place fruits into bowl. Add in sliced gelatin. Toss gently to combine. Ladle equal portions into bowls; garnish with toasted flax seeds. Serve.

Recipe #10 - Mushroom Sausages

Ingredients:

- 4 oz cremini mushrooms, sliced thinly
- 2 garlic cloves, sliced thinly
- 1/3 cup diced onion
- ½ tablespoon and 1 teaspoon olive oil
- ½ tablespoon maple syrup
- ½ tablespoon balsamic vinegar
- 2 tablespoons pecans or walnuts, chopped
- 1 tablespoon sunflower seeds
- ¾ cup dry breadcrumbs
- ½ teaspoon rubbed sage
- ½ teaspoon dried thyme
- ¼ teaspoon sea salt
- ¼ teaspoon freshly ground black pepper

Directions:

1. Heat a teaspoon of olive oil in a skillet over medium flame. Add the mushrooms and onion. Sauté until tender.
2. Add the sunflower seeds, nuts, herbs, garlic, salt, and pepper. Sauté until mixed well. Set aside and let cool.
3. Transfer the cooled mixture into a food processor. Add the maple syrup and balsamic vinegar. Blend until smooth.
4. Pour into a bowl and fold in the breadcrumbs. Mix well.

5. Divide the mixture into 4 pieces and shape into patties. Set aside.
6. Heat the remaining olive oil in a skillet over medium flame. Cook the patties until golden brown, about 3 minutes per side. Serve warm.

Recipe #11 - Sweet Potato Biscuits

Ingredients:

- 3 cups whole wheat flour
- 2/3 cup non-dairy milk
- ½ cup non-dairy butter
- 1 ½ cups pureed sweet potato
- ¾ teaspoon ground ginger
- 1 ¼ teaspoon ground cinnamon
- 3 teaspoons baking powder
- 2/3 teaspoon sea salt

Directions:

1. Set the oven to 400 degrees F. line a baking sheet with parchment paper.
2. Combine the dry ingredients in a bowl.
3. Cut the butter into the dry ingredients until the mixture looks crumbly.
4. Combine the pureed sweet potato with the milk in another bowl. Mix this into the dry ingredients.
5. Transfer the dough onto a lightly floured surface and knead well. Roll out with a rolling pin until ¾ inch thick. Cut into 24 pieces and arrange on the baking sheet, an inch apart.
6. Bake for 15 minutes, or until golden brown. Let cool at room temperature.

Recipe #12 – Spicy Scrambled Tofu

Ingredients:

- ½ tablespoon olive oil
- 1 small yellow onion, minced
- 1 garlic, minced
- ½ bell pepper, minced
- 8 oz extra firm tofu, drained and rinsed
- ¼ teaspoon cumin
- ¼ teaspoon turmeric
- ½ zucchini, chopped
- 1 small tomato, diced
- ½ jalapeno pepper, minced
- pinch of sea salt
- pinch of freshly ground black pepper

Directions:

1. Heat olive oil in skillet over medium flame. Sauté onion, garlic, and bell pepper until tender.
2. Crumble tofu into a bowl, and then add into the skillet. Sauté to mix.
3. Add the spices, zucchini, tomato, and jalapeno pepper. Sauté until golden and heated through.
4. Season to taste with salt and pepper.

Chapter 3 – Healthy Lunch Menus

Recipe #13 - Vegetarian Ragout

Ingredients:

- 1 ½ tablespoons olive oil
- 1 large eggplant, diced
- ½ small butternut squash, diced
- 1 small red onion, diced
- 2 garlic cloves, chopped
- ½ cup chopped tomatoes, juices reserved
- ¼ tablespoon tomato paste
- ½ cup canned chickpeas, rinsed and drained
- 1 green bell pepper, diced
- ½ teaspoon turmeric
- ½ teaspoon red chili powder
- ½ tsp fine sea salt
- freshly ground black pepper
- 3 fresh basil leaves

Directions:

1. Place a large saucepan over medium flame and heat through. Once hot, add the olive oil and swirl to coat.
2. Stir in the onion and sauté until translucent, then stir in the garlic and sauté until fragrant.

3. Add the squash, chickpeas, tomatoes, eggplants, bell pepper, tomato paste, turmeric, chili powder, and salt. Stir well and let simmer.
4. Cover and reduce to low flame. Cook for about 12 minutes, or until the vegetables are tender. Season to taste with black pepper.
5. Remove from heat and garnish with basil. Serve right away or pack for lunch on-the-go

Recipe #14 - Sweet Potato and Red Pepper Soup

Ingredients:

- 2 tablespoons olive oil
- 2 large red peppers
- 1 large sweet potato, cubed
- ½ cup onion, chopped
- 2 garlic cloves, minced
- ½ cup carrots, chopped
- ½ cup celery, chopped
- 2 ½ cups vegetable broth
- ½ cup coconut milk
- ¼ cup fresh sweet basil, julienned
- pinch of sea salt
- pinch of freshly ground black pepper

Directions:

1. Place the oven into the 375 degrees F.
2. Combine the onions and sweet potatoes on a baking sheet. Add the red peppers beside the mixture. Drizzle some of the olive oil over everything and toss well to coat.
3. Roast for 20 minutes, or until sweet potatoes are golden and peppers are tender and skins are wilted. Chop the roasted red peppers and set aside.
4. Place a pot over medium high flame and heat through. Once hot, add the olive oil and swirl to coat. Place the carrot, celery, and garlic into the pot

and sauté until carrot and celery are tender. Add the chopped roasted red peppers and sweet potato-onion mixture. Mix well.

5. Pour in the vegetable broth and coconut milk. Increase to high flame and bring to a boil. Once boiling, reduce to a simmer. Simmer, uncovered, for 10 minutes. Season to taste with salt and pepper, then turn off the heat and allow to cool slightly.

6. If desired, blend the soup using an immersion blender until the soup has reached a desired level of smoothness. Reheat over medium flame. Add the basil and stir to combine. Serve right away or pack for lunch on-the-go.

Recipe #15 - Cold Minty Avocado and Cucumber Soup

Ingredients:

- ½ cup coconut milk
- ½ small garlic clove, minced
- 2 small cucumber, chopped
- 1 small avocado, peeled
- 2 tablespoons freshly squeezed lime juice
- ¼ cup torn fresh mint leaves
- ¼ teaspoon cumin
- ½ teaspoon chopped green onion
- chilli powder
- pinch of sea salt
- pinch of freshly ground black pepper

Directions:

1. Place the avocado, lime juice, garlic, cucumber, cumin, and most of the mint leaves in a high power blender.
2. Cover and blend until pureed. Pour in the coconut milk and blend until smooth.
3. Season to taste with salt and pepper, then pour into bowls and add a dash of chili powder.
4. Scatter the green onion and remaining mint on top, then cover and refrigerate until chilled. Serve cold.

Recipe #16 - Avocado Edamame Spread

Ingredients:

- ¾ cup shelled edamame
- ½ small avocado, peeled
- 1 tablespoon lime juice, freshly squeezed
- 1 tablespoon olive oil
- 1 garlic clove
- 2 tablespoons fresh cilantro, chopped
- ¼ cup soy yogurt
- pinch of sea salt
- pinch of freshly ground black pepper

Directions:

1. Combine the cilantro and garlic in a food processor. Pulse until minced.
2. Add the remaining ingredients, except olive oil. Blend until smooth.
3. Gradually pour in the olive oil as you blend until mixture is smooth.
4. Pour into a container and top with chopped cilantro. Serve with leftover breakfast biscuits or vegetarian-friendly pretzels.

Recipe #17 - Egg Salad on Cucumbers

Ingredients:

- 2 large fresh cucumbers, sliced diagonally into ¼-inch thick medallions

For the Egg salad

- 6 large eggs, hardboiled, diced
- 1 large celery stalk, mince
- 3 tablespoons chives, mince
- 1 ½ tablespoons yellow mustard
- 1 teaspoon sweet pickle relish
- ¼ cup mayonnaise
- ⅛ teaspoon palm sugar, crumbled
- pinch of sea salt
- pinch of white pepper

Directions:

1. Combine salad ingredients in large bowl; mix well. Taste; adjust seasoning if needed. Chill salad for at least 30 minutes before serving.
2. Spread 1 heaping teaspoon of salad on cucumber disks.
3. Repeat step until you have 2 disks per person. Serve immediately.

Recipe #18 - Grilled Zucchini

Ingredients:

- 2 medium zucchini
- 2 tablespoons olive oil
- pinch of sea salt
- pinch of freshly ground black pepper

Directions:

1. Set the grill to high.
2. Slice the zucchini lengthwise using a mandolin or sharp knife. Place the zucchini in a bowl and add the olive oil. Season with salt and pepper. Toss to coat. Reduce grill to medium high.
3. Grill the zucchini for 2 minutes per side, turning only once. Place the zucchini on a plate lined with paper towels.

Recipe #19 - Avocado Pesto Pasta

Ingredients:

- vegetable pasta, any kind (example: Carrot Noodles – see recipe below)
- 1 large garlic clove
- 2 ½ tablespoons fresh basil leaves, chopped
- ½ teaspoon olive oil
- 1 tablespoon lemon juice, freshly squeezed
- ¼ teaspoon sea salt
- ½ small avocado, peeled
- pinch of sea salt
- pinch of freshly ground black pepper

Directions:

1. Cook the pasta based on the package instructions. Rinse over cold water, drain thoroughly, and set aside.
2. Meanwhile, combine the basil and garlic in a food processor. Pulse until pasty. Add the freshly squeezed lemon juice and avocado, then pulse until combined.
3. Gradually drizzle the olive oil into the pesto as you pulse, until everything is thoroughly mixed. Season to taste with salt and pepper.
4. Transfer the pasta into a serving bowl, then add the pesto. Toss well to coat, then serve right away.

Carrot Noodles

Ingredients:

- 2 large fresh carrots, tops removed, unpeeled, skin scrubbed clean
- pinch, generous sea salt

Directions:

1. Using vegetable peeler, scrape one side of carrot. Turn vegetable a quarter-way, and scrape that side too. Continue turning and scraping until most of the vegetable is processed. Discard the rest.
2. Place vegetables and salt into colander. Toss well to combine. Let these "sweat" and drain for 30 minutes. Shake off excess moisture.
3. Layer *coodles* (carrot noodles) on tea towel; roll tightly to remove more moisture and salt. Remove vegetable noodles from tea towel. Use as needed.

Recipe #20 - Veggie Coconut Curry

Ingredients:

- 1 tablespoon coconut oil
- 1 small broccoli head, chopped into florets
- 1 cup diced tomatoes, juices reserved
- 1 ½ cups coconut milk
- 1 cup chopped green beans
- 1 small onion, diced
- 2 garlic cloves, chopped
- ½ tablespoon ginger, minced
- 1 teaspoon crushed coriander
- ½ teaspoon turmeric
- ½ teaspoon all spice

Directions:

1. Place a soup pot over medium flame and heat through. Once hot, add the coconut oil and swirl to coat.
2. Add the onion, garlic, and ginger, then sauté until tender. Add the spices and sauté until fragrant.
3. Stir in the broccoli, green beans, and tomatoes. Mix well. Pour in the coconut milk and bring to a boil.
4. Once boiling, reduce to low flame and let simmer. Cover and cook for 8 to 10 minutes.
5. Uncover and cook for an additional 3 minutes, or until the sauce becomes slightly thickened. Serve.

Recipe #21 - Cauliflower Fettuccini

Ingredients:

- vegetable pasta (example: Swoodles – (Sweet Potato Noodles) – see recipe below)
- 2 ½ cups cauliflower florets, chopped
- 2 garlic cloves, minced
- ¼ tablespoon olive oil
- 2 ½ tablespoons nutritional yeast
- 2 ½ tablespoons non-dairy milk
- ¾ tablespoon lemon juice, freshly squeezed
- ¼ teaspoon onion powder
- ½ teaspoon sea salt
- pinch of freshly ground black pepper

Directions:

1. Cook the pasta based on the package instructions. Rinse over cold water, drain thoroughly, and set aside.
2. Place the cauliflower florets into a microwaveable bowl and add a few tablespoons of water. Microwave on high for 3 minutes, or until cauliflower is tender.
3. Place a skillet over medium flame and heat the olive oil. Swirl to coat, then sauté the garlic until fragrant.
4. Drain the cauliflower, then transfer to a food processor. Add the garlic, onion powder, milk, nutritional yeast, salt, and a pinch of pepper. Blend until smooth.

5. Transfer the pasta into a serving bowl, then add the sauce. Toss well to coat, then serve right away.

Swoodles (Sweet Potato Noodles)

Ingredients:

- 1 large fresh sweet potato, peeled, quartered lengthwise
- pinch, generous sea salt

Directions:

1. Using vegetable peeler, scrape cut side of sweet potato. Continue scraping until most of the vegetable is processed. Discard the rest.
2. Place vegetables and salt into colander. Toss well to combine. Let these "sweat" and drain for 30 minutes. Shake off excess moisture.
3. Layer *swoodles* on tea towel; roll tightly to remove more moisture and salt. Remove vegetable noodles from tea towel. Use as needed.

Recipe #22 - Vegan Mac 'n' Cheese

Ingredients:

- vegetable pasta (example: Proodles (Parsnip Noodles) see recipe below)
- 2 ½ tablespoons nutritional yeast
- 2 ½ tablespoons non-dairy butter
- ½ cup panko breadcrumbs
- 1 cup broccoli, steamed, chopped
- ½ cup sweet potato, diced
- ½ small carrot, diced
- ½ cup water
- ½ tablespoon miso paste
- ½ tablespoon lemon juice, freshly squeezed
- ½ tablespoon tahini
- ½ teaspoon Dijon mustard
- 2 tablespoons cashews, chopped
- ½ teaspoon sea salt

Directions:

1. Set the oven to 350 degrees F.
2. Cook the pasta based on the package instructions. Rinse over cold water, drain thoroughly, and set aside.
3. Combine the carrot and sweet potato into a saucepan and add the water. Place over high flame and boil for 8 minutes, or until tender.
4. Combine the remaining ingredients, except the breadcrumbs, pasta, broccoli, and carrot-sweet

potato mixture, in a food processor. Blend until smooth.

5. Combine all the ingredients in a casserole dish. Top with the panko breadcrumbs.
6. Bake for 15 minutes, or until top is golden brown. Best served warm.

Proodles (Parsnip Noodles)

Ingredients:

- 2 large fresh parsnip, tops removed, peeled
- pinch, generous sea salt

Directions:

1. Make deep scores spaced ⅛-inch apart on one side of parsnip. Using vegetable peeler, scrape this side of the vegetable repeatedly until you have a pile of noodles; make sure that you use long strokes. Discard the rest.
2. Mix and toss vegetables and salt into colander. Let vegetables "sweat" and drain for 30 minutes. Shake off excess moisture.
3. Layer *proodles* on tea towel; roll tightly to remove more moisture and salt. Remove vegetable noodles from tea towel. Use as needed.

Recipe #23 - Sweet and Sour Tofu with Veggies

Ingredients:

- ½ tablespoon coconut oil
- 7 oz extra firm tofu, sliced into strips
- 1 small yellow onion, chopped
- 1 garlic clove, minced
- 1 small green red pepper, chopped

For the Sweet and Sour Sauce:

- 1/3 cup pineapple chunks, juices reserved
- 2 ½ tablespoons brown rice vinegar
- 1 ½ tablespoons tomato paste
- ½ tablespoon soy sauce
- ½ tablespoon water
- ½ tablespoon corn starch

Directions:

1. Combine the water and corn starch for the sauce. Set aside.
2. In a saucepan, combine the soy sauce with the tomato paste, vinegar, and pineapple with the juices. Place over medium flame and bring to a simmer.
3. Once simmering, stir in the corn starch mixture. Simmer until thickened. Set aside.
4. Preheat the broiler. Place the rack in the upper third section of the oven.

45

5. Dip the tofu strips in the sweet and sour sauce, then arrange on a baking sheet. Broil for 5 minutes, then flip over and coat with more sauce. Broil for an additional 3 minutes. Repeat until the tofu is broiled.
6. Meanwhile, place a skillet over medium flame and heat through. Once hot, add the coconut oil and swirl to coat.
7. Add the onion and sauté until translucent. Add the garlic and sauté until fragrant. Add the bell pepper and sauté until tender.
8. Place sautéed vegetables on a serving dish. Add broiled tofu on top. Serve right away.

Recipe #24 - Barley and Butternut Squash Casserole

Ingredients:

- 1 tablespoon olive oil
- 1 tablespoon non-dairy butter
- ½ cup pearl barley
- 1 ¾ cups cubed butternut squash
- 1 garlic clove, minced
- ½ red onion minced
- 1 tablespoon whole wheat flour
- 1 cup non-dairy milk
- 1 teaspoon dried rosemary
- ½ cup vegetarian cheese, shredded
- Nutmeg
- ¼ teaspoon sea salt
- freshly ground black pepper

Directions:

1. Set the oven to 350 degrees F.
2. Combine the water and barley in a small pot, then place over high flame. Bring to a boil.
3. Once boiling, reduce to a simmer. Cover and boil for 15 to 20 minutes, or until the barley has fully absorbed the barley. Drain excess liquid and set aside.
4. Place a skillet over medium flame and heat through. Once heated, add the olive oil and swirl to coat.

5. Add the garlic and sauté until fragrant. Stir in the onion and sauté until translucent. Add the squash and sauté until tender. Place a saucepan over medium low flame and add the butter. Stir in the flour until pasty.
6. Add the milk and rosemary, then a dash of nutmeg. Season to taste with salt and pepper, then bring to a boil, whisking until thickened.
7. Turn off the heat. Stir in vegetarian cheese until thoroughly combined. Mix together the squash, barley and sauce in a baking dish. Seal with aluminum foil and bake for 15 minutes.
8. Uncover and set the oven to broil. Broil for 3 minutes, or until the casserole is golden brown. Set on a cooling rack. Let cool for 10 minutes, then serve.

Chapter 4 – Healthful Dinner Meals

Recipe #25 - Veggie Pita

Ingredients:

- 1 teaspoon non-dairy butter
- ½ cup broccoli, thinly sliced
- ½ cup cauliflower, thinly sliced
- ½ onion, thinly sliced
- 2 tomatoes, chopped
- 4 tablespoons non-dairy cheddar cheese
- 1 whole vegetarian pita pocket bread, halved
- italian seasoning

Directions:

1. Combine the butter, broccoli, and cauliflower in a microwaveable bowl.
2. Cover the bowl with parchment paper, then microwave for 2 minutes on high.
3. Carefully remove the bowl from the microwave and add the tomatoes, cheese, and onions. Season with a pinch of Italian seasoning.
4. Spoon the mixture into the pita bread, then serve or pack for lunch on-the-go.

Recipe #26 - Sweet Potato and Corn Tortilla Rolls

Ingredients:

- ½ tablespoon olive oil
- 1 ½ cups diced sweet potatoes
- 1 ½ cups diced tomatoes
- ½ cup corn kernels
- ½ red bell pepper, diced
- 1 ½ teaspoon cumin
- 2 whole wheat tortillas

Directions:

1. Set the oven to 400 degrees F.
2. Spread the diced sweet potatoes on a baking sheet, then drizzle the olive oil on top. Sprinkle the cumin over them, then toss well to coat.
3. Bake the sweet potatoes for 20 minutes.
4. Meanwhile, place a non-stick skillet over medium flame and heat through. Once hot, add corn, bell pepper, and tomatoes. Simmer for 10 minutes.
5. Once the sweet potatoes are baked, divide them between the tortillas. Heap the black bean and corn mixture on top, then roll up securely.
6. Serve right away or pack for lunch on-the-go.

Recipe #27 - Lemon Garlic Broccoli

Ingredients:

- 1 ½ tablespoons olive oil
- 1 broccoli head, chopped into florets
- 1 garlic clove, minced
- ¼ teaspoon lemon juice, freshly squeezed
- pinch of sea salt
- pinch of freshly ground black pepper

Directions:

1. Set the oven to 400 degrees F.
2. Spread the chopped broccoli on a baking sheet. Drizzle the olive oil and season to taste with salt and pepper. Toss well to coat.
3. Sprinkle with freshly squeezed lemon juice. Roast for 15 minutes. Best served warm.

Recipe #28 - Coconut and Ginger Pasta

Ingredients:

- vegetable pasta (example: Prydles (Purple Yam Noodles) see recipe below)
- 1 cup spinach leaves, dried
- ½ cup Swiss chard, dried
- ½ tablespoon olive oil
- 2 small garlic cloves, minced
- 1 ½ tablespoons grated fresh ginger
- 8 oz coconut milk
- 1 ½ teaspoons lemon juice, freshly squeezed
- red pepper flakes
- pinch of sea salt
- pinch of freshly ground black pepper

Directions:

1. Cook the pasta based on the package instructions. Rinse over cold water, drain thoroughly, and set aside.
2. Meanwhile, place a saucepan over medium flame and heat the olive oil. Stir in the garlic and ginger until fragrant. Add the stevia and coconut milk. Mix well.
3. Season with red pepper flakes, salt, and pepper. Let simmer, stirring frequently.
4. Add the spinach and Swiss chard, then cover the saucepan. Let simmer for about 4 minutes. Turn off

the heat and let cool, then pour into a blender or food processor. Blend until creamy.

5. Transfer the pasta into a serving bowl, then add the sauce. Toss well to coat, then serve right away.

Prydles (Purple Yam Noodles)

Ingredients:

- 1 large purple yam, quartered lengthwise
- pinch, generous sea salt
- water, for soaking/rinsing

Directions:

1. Make deep scores spaced ⅛-inch apart on one side of yam. Using vegetable peeler, scrape cut side of vegetable repeatedly until you have a pile of noodles; make sure that you use long strokes. Discard the rest.
2. Submerge vegetable noodles in water for 20 minutes, and then rinse vigorously until water becomes clear. Mix and toss vegetables and salt into colander. Let vegetables "sweat" and drain for 30 minutes. Shake off excess moisture.
3. Layer *prydles* on tea towel; roll tightly to remove more moisture and salt. Remove vegetable noodles from tea towel. Use as needed.

Recipe #29 - Savory Mushroom Stroganoff

Ingredients:

- 3 tablespoons olive oil
- 6 oz shiitake mushrooms, chopped
- 18 oz large Portobello mushroom caps, chopped
- 1 large onion, chopped
- 1 ½ cups frozen baby onions, defrosted
- 4 garlic cloves, crushed
- 1 ½ cups coconut cream or vegan sour cream
- 3 tablespoons soy sauce
- ¾ cup vegetable broth
- 3 tablespoons fresh flat leaf parsley, chopped
- pinch of sea salt
- pinch of freshly ground black pepper

Directions:

1. Place a large saucepan over medium flame and heat through. Once hot, add 2 tablespoons of oil and swirl to coat.
2. Add the mushrooms and sauté for 6 minutes, or until tender. Transfer to a bowl and set aside.
3. Pour the remaining oil into the saucepan and swirl to coat. Stir in the chopped onion until translucent. Add the garlic and sauté until fragrant. Return the mushrooms to the pan and sauté with the onion and garlic.

4. Pour in the soy sauce and mix well. Add the vegetable broth and stir. Bring to a simmer, then add the baby onions.
5. Cook for 3 minutes, or until the stock has reduced to half its original volume and the baby onions are heated through.
6. Reduce to low flame and stir in the cream. Sprinkle the parsley on top and serve right away.

Recipe #30 - Cabbage Lasagna

Ingredients:

- 1 large cabbage head
- 1 cup canned corn kernels, rinsed and drained
- 3 cups thinly sliced mushrooms
- 3 large eggplants, diced
- 3 cups grated non-dairy mozzarella or cheddar cheese
- ¾ cup chopped black olives
- 1 ½ cups chopped tomatoes
- ¾ cup vegetable broth
- 4 tablespoons olive oil
- 6 sprigs fresh basil

Directions:

1. Set the oven to 375 degrees F.
2. Carefully remove the cabbage leaves, making sure to retain their original shape. These will be your "lasagna pasta."
3. Place a large non-stick skillet over medium flame and heat through. Once hot, add 3 tablespoons of olive oil and swirl to coat. Sauté the garlic until fragrant, then add the mushrooms and eggplants. Sauté until tender.
4. Pour in the chopped tomatoes with their juices and the vegetable broth. Mix well and simmer until eggplant is tender. Simmer until sauce is thickened.

5. Lightly coat a large baking dish with the remaining olive oil. Create a single layer of cabbage leaves. Ladle the vegetable mixture on top, then scatter some olives and corn kernels over it.
6. Add another layer of cabbage leaves, followed by a layer of the cheese. Ladle on the vegetable mixture. Keep repeating until the last layer is cheese.
7. Bake for 20 minutes in the oven, then set on a cooling rack for 15 minutes. To serve, cut and garnish with fresh basil. Best served warm.

Recipe #31 - Savory Tofu-Seitan Loaf

Ingredients:

- 7 oz firm tofu
- 1 lb ground seitan
- ½ oz dry onion soup mix
- ½ cup panko breadcrumbs
- 2 ½ tablespoons minced bell pepper
- 1 egg or egg substitute
- ½ tsp Dijon mustard

Directions:

1. Set the oven to 350 degrees F.
2. Combine the tofu, ground seitan, and panko breadcrumbs in a bowl. Add the green bell pepper and egg or egg substitute. Mix well.
3. Add the dry onion soup mix and mix well, then pack the mixture into a bread pan.
4. Put yellow mustard in a bowl, then pour over the mixture. Bake for 30 minutes, or until firm and golden brown. Best served warm.

Recipe #32 - Hearty Mushroom Chili

Ingredients:

- 1 tablespoon olive oil
- ¾ cup onion, diced
- 1 tablespoon garlic, minced
- 6 oz chopped cremini mushrooms
- 7 oz canned fire-roasted crushed tomatoes with green chilies
- 1/3 cup green bell pepper, diced
- 1/3 cup red bell pepper, diced
- ½ jalapeno pepper, seeded and minced
- 1 tablespoon garlic, minced
- 1 teaspoon chili powder
- 1 teaspoon mashed chipotle chili in adobo sauce
- ¾ teaspoon cumin
- ¾ teaspoon dried oregano
- 1/3 cup water
- 2 ½ tablespoons fresh cilantro, chopped
- 1/3 teaspoon sea salt
- ¼ teaspoon freshly ground black pepper

Directions:

1. Place a pot over medium flame and heat through. Once hot, add the olive oil and swirl to coat.
2. Add the onion and sauté until translucent. Stir in the bell pepper and jalapeno. Sauté until tender.
3. Stir in the garlic and mushrooms, then sauté until mushrooms are tender. Stir in the chipotle chili,

chili powder, oregano, and cumin. Sauté until fragrant.

4. Add tomatoes, salt, black pepper, cilantro, and water. Let simmer, then reduce to low flame.

5. Cover and simmer for 12 minutes or until the sauce thickens. Best served warm.

Recipe #33 - Seitan Shawarma

Ingredients:

- ½ lb seitan
- 1 ½ teaspoon nutritional yeast
- ¼ cup water
- ½ onion, diced
- 1 tablespoon apple cider vinegar
- 1 ½ tablespoons lemon juice, freshly squeezed
- 1 teaspoon Dijon mustard
- ¼ teaspoon ground ginger
- ¼ teaspoon cumin
- pinch of sea salt
- pinch of freshly ground black pepper

Directions:

1. Slice the seitan into thin strips. Set aside.
2. Boil the water in a small saucepan, then stir the nutritional yeast into it. Add the remaining ingredients, except the seitan, and mix well.
3. Pour the mixture over the seitan, then turn to coat. Refrigerate for 2 hours to marinate.
4. To cook, place a non-stick skillet over medium high flame and heat through. Once hot, add the seitan strips and cook for 5 minutes per side. Best served hot.

Recipe #34 - Vegetarian Moroccan Stew

Ingredients:

- 2 tablespoons olive oil
- 1 small onion, thinly sliced
- 1 garlic clove, crushed
- 28 oz extra firm tofu, sliced into large cubes
- 1/3 cup vegetable broth
- ½ tablespoon tomato paste
- ½ teaspoon sea salt
- ¼ teaspoon freshly ground black pepper

For the Spice Blend:

- ¼ teaspoon cinnamon
- ¼ teaspoon coriander
- ¼ teaspoon paprika
- ¼ teaspoon cumin
- ½ teaspoon ground ginger

Directions:

1. Combine the spice blend and mix well.
2. Place a heavy saucepan over medium flame and heat through. Once hot, add the oil and swirl to coat. Add the cubed tofu and cook carefully until browned all over. Transfer to a plate lined with paper towels and set aside.
3. Using the same saucepan, sauté the onion until translucent. Add the garlic and sauté until fragrant.

Pour in the broth and stir in the remaining ingredients. Reduce to low flame and simmer for 15 minutes.
4. Add the cooked tofu and mix carefully. Transfer to a serving dish and serve right away.

Recipe #35 - Festive Vegetarian Pasta

Ingredients:

- vegetable pasta (example: Toodles (Taro Noodles) see recipe below)
- 1 carrot, sliced thinly
- 1 small zucchini, sliced thinly
- 1 small yellow summer squash, sliced thinly
- 1 small red bell pepper, julienned
- ¼ cup green onion, chopped
- ½ cup asparagus, thinly sliced
- ¼ cup peas
- ¼ cup green onions, chopped
- 1 ½ tablespoons nutritional yeast
- 1 tablespoon fresh dill, chopped
- 1 tablespoon non-dairy butter
- ½ tablespoon lemon juice, freshly squeezed
- 1/3 cup vegetable broth
- 2 ½ tablespoon chopped sun-dried tomatoes
- 1/3 teaspoon sea salt
- ¼ teaspoon freshly ground black pepper
- olive oil

Directions:

1. Prepare the farfalle pasta based on package directions. Drain thoroughly; do not rinse. Set aside. Place a large, non-stick skillet over medium flame and heat through. Once hot, add enough olive oil to coat the base.

2. Add the summer squash, zucchini, bell pepper, carrot, asparagus, sun-dried tomatoes, and ¼ cup vegetable broth. Mix well. Simmer, stirring constantly, until the vegetables are tender. Add the peas and green onion, then sauté until mixed and heated through.
3. Stir in the farfalle pasta, parsley, basil, nutritional yeast, butter, lemon juice, and remaining vegetable broth. Season to taste with salt and pepper, then mix well.
4. Transfer to a serving bowl and serve right away.

Toodles (Taro Noodles)

Ingredients:

- 1 large fresh taro, quartered lengthwise
- pinch, generous sea salt
- water, for soaking/rinsing

Directions:

1. Using vegetable peeler, scrape cut side of taro. Continue scraping until most of the vegetable is processed. Discard the rest.
2. Submerge vegetable noodles in water for 20 minutes, and then rinse vigorously until water becomes clear. Drain well. Place vegetables and salt into colander. Toss well to combine. Let these "sweat" and drain for 30 minutes. Shake off excess moisture.

3. Layer *toodles* on tea towel; roll tightly to remove more moisture and salt. Remove vegetable noodles from tea towel. Use as needed.

Recipe #36 - Hearty French Tofu and Vegetable Stew

Ingredients:

- 24 oz extra firm tofu, sliced into large cubes
- ¾ tablespoon olive oil
- 1 small onion, quartered
- 2 garlic cloves, crushed
- ¾ tablespoon non-dairy butter
- 1 turnip, cubed
- 1 carrot, cubed
- ½ head cabbage, shredded
- ¼ teaspoon dried thyme
- ¼ teaspoon dried basil
- ¼ teaspoon dried rosemary
- 1 bay leaf
- pinch of sea salt
- pinch of freshly ground black pepper

Directions:

1. Place a heavy skillet over medium flame and heat through. Once hot, add the oil and butter and swirl to coat. Add the tofu and cook until browned all over. Transfer to a plate.
2. Place the carrot, turnip, and onion into the same skillet and sauté until browned, scraping the bottom to loosen any browned bits.
3. Add a bit of water and simmer for 10 minutes or until the root vegetables are tender and the water

has evaporated. Add more water, if needed. Stir the cabbage into the skillet and mix well. Add the thyme, basil, rosemary, and basil.

4. Season to taste with salt and pepper, then add the cooked tofu. Carefully mix well. Serve right away.

Chapter 5 – Eat Fat Get Thin Snacks and Desserts

Recipe #37 - Balsamic Blackberry Jam

Ingredients:

- 3 tablespoons balsamic vinegar
- 2½ pounds frozen blackberries, thawed
- 1 cup raw organic honey
- ¼ cup water
- ½ large lemon, freshly juiced

Directions:

1. Place ingredients in large heavy-bottomed saucepan set over medium heat; boil. Reduce heat to lowest setting.
2. Using potato masher, mash berries; cook until most of liquid has evaporated, stirring frequently. Turn off heat.
3. Cool completely to room temperature before storing in airtight container; use as needed.

Recipe #38 - Thyme Berry Jam

Ingredients:

- 10 sprigs fresh thyme, whole
- 1 cup frozen blueberries, thawed
- 1 cup frozen cranberries, thawed
- 1 cup frozen loganberry, thawed
- 1 cup raw organic honey
- ¼ cup water
- ½ large lemon, fresh juiced, pips removed

Directions:

1. Except for thyme sprigs, place ingredients in large heavy-bottomed saucepan set over medium heat; boil. Reduce heat to lowest setting.
2. Using potato masher, mash berries; add in thyme sprigs. Cook until most liquid has evaporated, stirring frequently. Turn off heat. Fish out and discard thyme.
3. Cool completely to room temperature before storing in airtight container; use as needed.

Recipe #39 - Fried Asparagus

Ingredients:

- coconut oil for shallow frying

Fried asparagus

- 3 large eggs, whisked
- 1 pound, thick-stemmed green asparagus, sliced into 3 inch long slivers
- 1 pound, thick-stemmed white asparagus, sliced into 3 inch long slivers
- 1 cup almond meal
- 1 cup almond flour, finely milled
- pinch of sea salt
- dash of cumin powder

Directions:

1. Pour small amount of oil into non-stick skillet set over medium heat. Dredge fruit in almond flour first, and then into eggs, and into almond meal; shake off excess starch.
2. Carefully slide breaded pieces into oil; fry until crisp and golden, flipping often. Drain on paper towels. Season with sea salt; serve.

Recipe #40 - Fried Mushrooms and Onions Fritters

Ingredients:

- coconut oil for shallow frying
- 2 large eggs, whisked
- 2 large sweet onions, julienned
- 2 cups almond meal
- 2cups almond flour, finely milled
- 1 pound enoki mushrooms, bottoms trimmed
- pinch of sea salt
- dried oregano to taste

Directions:

1. Pour small amount of oil into non-stick skillet set over medium heat. Toss enoki mushrooms and julienned onions into almond flour until well-coated. Shake off excess starch.
2. Take a generous pinch of both mushrooms and onions, and dunk these as one large piece into whisked egg, and then into the almond meal. Carefully place on skillet; fry on both sides until golden. Drain on paper towels.
3. Repeat step until all mushrooms and onions are cooked. Season with sea salt and dried oregano; serve.

Recipe #41 - Herbed Cashew Cheese Stuffed Zucchini Blossoms

Ingredients:

- 10 large zucchini blossoms, preferably with 2 inches of stems still attached
- coconut oil for deep frying

Batter

- 2 cups coconut flour, finely milled
- 2 cups coconut water, sugar-free
- 1½ teaspoon sea salt

Herbed cheese filling

- 2 cups raw cashew nuts
- filtered water for soaking
- 4 tablespoons nutritional yeast
- 2 teaspoons garlic powder
- 2 teaspoons olive oil
- ¼ teaspoon dried oregano powder
- ¼ teaspoon Spanish paprika powder
- 1 large lemon, freshly juiced

Directions:

1. For herbed cheese filling: place cashew nuts in bowl. Pour in filtered water to fully submerge nuts;

soak overnight. Rinse and drain. Pour cashew nuts and remaining filling ingredients in blender; process until smooth.

2. Spoon equal portions into zucchini blossoms (approximately 1 heaping teaspoon); gently twist tips of blossoms to seal. Freeze flowers until ready to cook.

3. Half-fill deep fryer with coconut oil; set at high heat.

4. Mix batter ingredients in a bowl until lumps disappear; dip stuffed blossoms until lightly coated. Drain off excess batter. Slide stuffed blossoms into hot oil and fry until golden. These will cook in less than 3 minutes. Drain on paper towels. Serve 3 stuffed blossoms per person.

Recipe #42 - Mushrooms Stuffed with Cauliflower

Ingredients:

- 2 dozen large fresh portabella or shiitake mushrooms, stems minced
- ¼ cup fresh parsley, minced

For the Cauliflower filling

- 3 tablespoons coconut oil
- 2 tablespoons fresh parsley, minced
- 2 large garlic cloves, grated
- 1 large white onion, minced
- 1 head cauliflower, minced
- ¼ cup coconut vinegar
- dash of red pepper flakes
- pinch of sea salt
- pinch of black pepper

Directions:

1. Preheat oven to 400°F/200°C. Line 2 rimmed baking sheets with aluminum foil; lightly grease with coconut oil.
2. Pour oil into non-stick skillet set over medium heat; sauté garlic, onion, and pepper flakes until limp and transparent.
3. Stir in remaining cauliflower filling ingredients; cook mixture down until liquids has evaporated

75

completely, and cauliflower browns a little. Remove from heat. Cool slightly before spooning into mushroom caps.

4. Set filled mushrooms on baking sheets; tent loosely with aluminum foil. Bake for 15 to 20 minutes, or until mushrooms are fork tender.

5. Remove from heat; place mushrooms on individual plates. Garnish with parsley if using. Serve.

Recipe #43 - Zucchini Rolls with Herbed Almond Cream Cheese

Ingredients:

Cheese filling

- 1 cup blanched almonds
- filtered water for soaking
- fresh boiled water for blanching
- 1 teaspoon sea salt
- 1 teaspoon coconut vinegar
- ½ teaspoon basil leaves, minced
- ½ teaspoon parsley leaves, minced
- dash of onion powder

Zucchini rolls

- 3 small zucchini, using a vegetable peeler, shave off into wide slivers

Directions:

1. For cheese filling: place almonds in bowl. Pour in filtered water to fully submerge nuts; soak overnight. Rinse and drain. Blanch nuts with fresh boiled water. Steep for 5 minutes; drain.
2. Process almonds and remaining cream cheese ingredients in blender until smooth; place cheese in fridge until it sets.

3. Place parchment paper on flat surface; line zucchini slivers side by side. Place small amount of cream cheese mixture on top.
4. Roll up filled zucchini slivers, securing each with toothpicks. Serve 4 roll-ups per person.

Recipe #44 - Avocado and Pomegranate Salad with Cinnamon Vinaigrette

Ingredients:

Vinaigrette

- ½ cup extra virgin olive oil
- ¼ cup vinegar
- 1 large leek, minced
- 1 large Serrano chili, minced
- ½ teaspoon cinnamon powder
- pinch of sea salt
- pinch of black pepper

Salad

- 1 pound iceberg lettuce, torn
- ½ pound baby spinach leaves, torn
- ½ pound fresh strawberries, quartered
- 1 large avocado, cubed
- ¼ cup cashew nuts, freshly toasted

Directions:

1. Whisk dressing/vinaigrette ingredients until salt dissolves. Place salad ingredients in a bowl; season with half of dressing. Toss to combine; spoon salad into plates.
2. Season with more vinaigrette only if needed; serve.

Recipe #45 - Endive Salad with Strawberry Vinaigrette

Ingredients:

Dressing

- 2 cups frozen strawberries, thawed
- 2 tablespoons apple cider vinegar
- ¼ cup extra virgin olive oil
- ⅛ cup lemon juice, freshly squeezed
- pinch of sea salt
- pinch of black pepper

Salad

- 1 pound frisée lettuce, torn
- 1 pound Belgian endive lettuce, torn
- ½ pound escarole lettuce, torn
- ¼ pound frozen strawberries, thawed, quartered

Directions:

Whisk dressing/vinaigrette ingredients until salt dissolves. Place salad ingredients in a bowl; season with half of dressing. Toss to combine; spoon salad into plates.

Season with more vinaigrette only if needed; serve.

Recipe #46 - Green Salad with Eggs and Dried Herb Vinaigrette

Ingredients:

- 6 small eggs, soft-boiled, peeled

For the Vinaigrette

- 2 large garlic cloves, grated
- 1 large leeks, minced
- ½ teaspoon dried basil
- ½ teaspoon dried oregano
- ½ teaspoon dried rosemary
- ½ teaspoon dried thyme
- ½ cup coconut olive oil, melted
- ⅛ cup coconut vinegar
- ⅛ cup lime juice, freshly squeezed
- pinch of sea salt
- pinch of black pepper

For the Salad

- 1 head iceberg lettuce, torn
- ½ pound baby beet tops, torn
- ½ pound baby spinach leaves, torn

Directions:

1. To prepare vinaigrette: vigorously rub dried herbs between your palms to shred. Place these along with remaining vinaigrette ingredients into bottle with tight fitting lid; shake well.
2. Place salad ingredients in a bowl; season with half of vinaigrette. Toss to combine. Spoon salad into plates and top each off with soft-boiled egg.
3. Break eggs so yolks drip into the greens. Add more vinaigrette only if needed. Serve.

Recipe #47 - Rainbow Fruit Salad

Ingredients:

- 2 cups dark or purple colored seedless grapes, halved
- 2cups red watermelon, cubed into bite-sized pieces
- 2 cups yellow watermelon, cubed into bite-sized pieces
- 1 cup frozen blueberries, thawed
- 2 large kiwi fruits, quartered
- 1 large pomegranate, juiced
- 1 can mandarin oranges, drained
- honey to taste

Directions:

- Except for honey, place remaining ingredients (including pomegranate juice) in a bowl; toss gently to combine.
- Spoon equal amounts into individual serving bowls; drizzle small amount of honey on top of just before serving.

Recipe #48 - Green Noodle Salad with Spicy Raspberry Dressing

Ingredients:

- 1 cup frozen raspberries, thawed, halved

For the Dressing

- 4 large frozen raspberries, thawed, minced
- 1 large jalapeño pepper, deseeded, minced
- 1 large Thai green chili, deseeded, minced
- 1 teaspoon Dijon mustard
- ½ cup extra virgin olive oil
- ⅛ cup apple cider vinegar
- ⅛ cup raspberry vinegar
- pinch of sea salt
- pinch of black pepper

For the Salad

- 2 heads green oak leaf lettuce, sliced into 2-inch long slivers,
- head arugula, sliced into 2-inch long slivers
- 1 large cucumber, processed into flat noodles using *spiralizer* or vegetable peeler
- 1 small zucchini, processed into flat noodles using *spiralizer* or vegetable peeler

Directions:

1. Place dressing ingredients into bottle with tight fitting lid; shake until dressing emulsifies.
2. Place salad ingredients in a bowl; season with half of vinaigrette. Toss to combine.
3. Spoon salad into plates and top each off with equal amounts of raspberries. Season with more dressing if desired; serve.

Recipe #49 - Breaded Baby Corn

Ingredients:

- 1 pound baby corn, silks removed
- 1 cup almond flour, finely milled
- 1 cup almond milk
- 1 cup *panko* breading
- olive oil or coconut oil for shallow frying
- pinch of kosher salt
- pinch of white pepper
- dash of Spanish paprika

Directions:

1. Pour oil into non-stick skillet set over medium heat. Meanwhile, place flour, milk, and *panko* breading into 3 different shallow bowls.
2. Dredge baby corn in flour first, and then into the milk; coat generously with *panko* breading.
3. Repeat step until all baby corn are breaded. Fry these in oil until crisp and golden brown. Drain on paper towels. Just before serving, season well with salt and paprika.

Recipe #50 - Super Baked Tempeh Hash

Ingredients:

- 8 oz tempeh, crumbled
- 2 tablespoons extra virgin olive oil
- ¼ cup diced red onion
- 1 garlic clove, minced
- ¼ cup kale, chopped
- 1 small red bell pepper, diced
- ½ cup Yukon Gold potatoes, grated
- 2 tablespoons pumpkin seeds
- 2 tablespoons nutritional yeast
- 1 tablespoon soy sauce
- ½ tablespoon apple cider vinegar
- ½ teaspoon paprika
- ½ teaspoon mustard powder
- ½ teaspoon onion powder
- ½ teaspoon freshly ground black pepper

Directions:

1. Set the oven to 350 degrees F. Line a baking sheet with aluminum foil.
2. Combine the spices, pepper, olive oil, vinegar, and soy sauce in a bowl. Add the diced onion, garlic, potato, bell pepper, kale, nutritional yeast, pumpkin seeds, and tempeh. Mix well.
3. Spread the mixture on the prepared baking sheet. Bake for 20 to 25 minutes. Slice and serve.

Conclusion

Thank you for purchasing this book!

I hope this book was able to help you know more about the Eat Fat Get Thin Diet as well as the many recipes that you can make in order to eliminate cravings, start losing weight and reverse diseases brought by an unhealthy lifestyle.

The next step is to try the recipes yourself and experiment on making other dishes using fresh produce as your main ingredients. Start eating good fat and clean, whole food. It is never too late for that big shift.

Finally, if you enjoyed this book, then I'd like to ask you for a favor, would you be kind enough to leave a review for this book on Amazon? It'd be greatly appreciated!

Thank you and good luck!

Made in the USA
Coppell, TX
02 August 2022

ISBN 9781537281445

9 781537 281445

AN OLD-FASHIONED
COUP

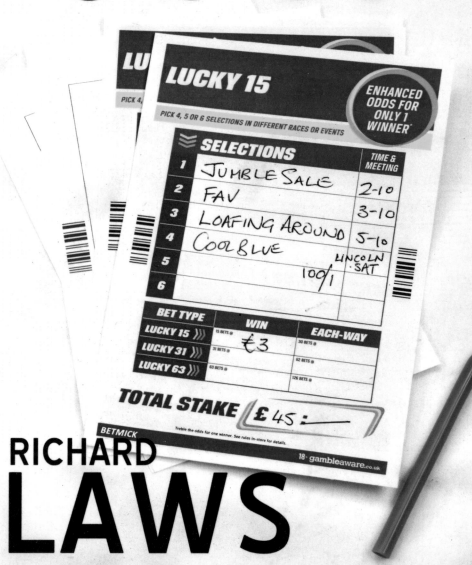

RICHARD
LAWS